Submissive Training

23 Things You Must Know About How To Be A Submissive. A Must Read For Any Woman In A BDSM Relationship

Elizabeth Cramer
Copyright© 2013 by Elizabeth Cramer

Copyright© 2013 Elizabeth Cramer
All Rights Reserved.

Warning: The unauthorized reproduction or distribution of this copyrighted work is illegal. No part of this book may be scanned, uploaded or distributed via internet or other means, electronic or print without the author's permission. Criminal copyright infringement without monetary gain is investigated by the FBI and is punishable by up to 5 years in federal prison and a fine of $250,000. (http://www.fbi.gov/ipr/). Please purchase only authorized electronic or print editions and do not participate in or encourage the electronic piracy of copyrighted material.

Publisher: Living Plus Healthy Publishing

ISBN-13: 978-1493760169

ISBN-10: 1493760165

Disclaimer

The Publisher has strived to be as accurate and complete as possible in the creation of this book. While all attempts have been made to verify information provided in this publication, the Publisher assumes no responsibility for errors, omissions, or contrary interpretation of the subject matter herein. Any perceived slights of specific persons, peoples, or organizations are unintentional.

This book is not intended for use as a source of legal, business, accounting or financial advice. All readers are advised to seek services of competent professionals in the legal, business, accounting, and finance fields.

The information in this book is not intended or implied to be a substitute for professional medical advice, diagnosis or treatment. All content contained in this book is for general information purposes only. Always consult your healthcare provider before carrying on any health program.

Table of Contents

Introduction 3
Section I: What You Will Learn 7
   1. Your Identity 7
   2. Your Value 10
   3. Proper Names 12
   4. Proper Language 16
   5. Proper Clothing 18
   6. Proper Graces 22
   7. Proper Postures 24
   8. The Value of Silence 27
   9. Asking Permission 30
   10. Attentiveness 33
   11. Gratitude 36
   12. Submitting Your Body for Inspection 39
   13. Submitting Your Body for Correction. 42
   14. Submitting Your Body for Ownership 46
   15. Submitting Your Body for Sexual Service 48
   16. Submitting Your Mouth for Your Master's Use .. 50
   17. Submitting Your Vagina for Your Master's Use . 52
   18. Submitting Your Ass for Sexual Service 54

Section II: How You Will Learn It 57

    19. Through Obedience 57

    20. Through Objectification 60

    21. Through Humiliation... 62

    22. By Repetition And Ritual....................................... 65

    23. By Affection.. 67

Conclusion... 69

Introduction

At the point you begin training as a submissive partner or slave, you have already taken a number of foundational steps along this journey. Hopefully you have identified your submissive inner nature and taken some time to explore the meaning submitting to another person has in your life.

Note: If you are completely new to the BDSM world, please read Vol. 1 and 2 of this "Women's Guide to BDSM" series:

BDSM Primer - A Woman's Guide to BDSM - Fetishes, Roles, Rituals, Protocols, Safety, & More, and *Care and Nurture for the Submissive - A Must Read for Any Woman in a BDSM Relationship*,

available at all major book retailers.

Most women look at blogs, books or fetish sites to learn the language, expectations and general way-of-life submissive women experience. However, nothing will prepare you for a life of submission in the same way as your formal training. Training isn't just a "good idea" when it comes to creating a BDSM relationship. It is essential.

Rushing into a relationship or service contract with a Dom without training puts the future of your time together at risk. All of the arguments, resistance, misunderstandings and hurt feelings that go with a new submissive's experiences can be eradicated by a period designated for learning, listening, trial and error.

Even if you have been with a previous Dom you will need to go through an abbreviated training time to ensure your patterns and understandings match one another. Training is a way to "get in the same rhythm" and find the perfect groove.

Couples who have previously experienced submission via email or a long distance relationship require as much training as a new arrangement. Talking about serving is much different than actually experiencing a submissive's life. There is a lot more downtime, accountability, and exhaustion than anything you will experience online.

This guide is designed to help you know what to expect when you go through training with a new Dom. Every couple is unique and every Dom may have different ways of teaching you the systems of service he prefers. However, these are the basics all trained subs and slaves learn and employ in daily life.

A slave and a sub are different in technical aspects, yet they are similar enough in their service that this guide will cover features for both and the words may be used interchangeably.

This guide has also been written to assume a 24/7 living situation for the Dom and sub. If you do not live with your Dom you'll find these same elements can be employed on a weekend or session basis just as easily. Although training does not lend itself to online Doms or virtual slavery, the thoughts and motivations behind the elements of training will still be useful as you construct your relationship.

This guide is divided into two sections:

1. What you will learn.
2. How you will learn it.

Finally, a note about protocol. There are a variety of levels of protocol depending on the couple practicing BDSM and their living situation. A couple may be a 24/7 high protocol couple where nudity, formality of language, and ritual is practiced at all times.

Likewise, a couple with children who enjoys BDSM on a session or "when the kids are at school" basis may use informal protocol for daily life (always showing respect, but not wearing a collar) and employ higher protocol when they are alone.

Because training often aims at the highest standard of expectation, this guide is written with medium-high protocol in mind. It is always best to train with the highest protocol possible. It is easier to train for a lot then be allowed to do less, than be trained for a little and be expected to do more.

Section I: What You Will Learn

1. Your Identity

Central to your training is the primary understanding that you are becoming, through thoughts, words and actions who you have always been on the inside. The purpose of training is to scrape away the roles, myths and conventions of society within the context of your relationship and replace it with the reality of your core being.

Training does not make you someone new; it brings out the person you already are. Although your life and attitude most definitely will change, do not go into training expecting it to make you a different person. It will give you the tools to become the person you were always meant to be.

That is why training should not be undertaken lightly or without a full commitment of service to your Master. You are learning to serve, live and love him as his slave or submissive partner for as long as you both desire.

In the larger social structure of western culture, women are taught via media, family and school that they are equal to men in all areas. Women are encouraged to develop and find their identity based on the scope of individualism. Who you are as a singular being is what matters and what defines you. As such, women are taught to measure themselves by their accomplishments at school, at work, as a spouse, parent, housekeeper, etc.

In training you will learn your identity is not made of your individual achievements (although they are important) but your relational context with your Dom. You are his. That is the core of your identity. That is who you are and how you will define all the other roles and lenses you look through.

Your identity as an owned and beloved submissive to your Master will take time to evolve as the core of your being. You are no longer a business executive. You are his submissive who works as a business executive. You are no longer an athlete. You are his submissive who is athletic.

In time, looking through the world through the lens of his eyes will become second nature to you and you will marvel that you ever enjoyed the surroundings of your life without his pride, love and ownership of you being a motivating factor.

It is a source of pride to the submissive that when people look at her they are seeing a couple. A Dom whose pride and dignity is reflected in the obedience, adoration and attention of his sub is one who is respected, and rightfully so.

The bonus for you, of course, is that you do not have to suffer the pressure or loneliness that comes from having to do everything, be responsible for everything and assure everything by yourself. In the harbor of your relationship your Master surrounds you with love, affirmation, inspiration, motivation and pride.

Being a submissive partner of a Master who has trained and sustained you means you are never alone. You are equal in your ability to consent to your submission. You are empowered with the ability to offer your Master all that you have, say, do and accomplish. You are his.

2. Your Value

BDSM is more than just sex and spankings. It goes much deeper than the physical, sexual reality of the situation. In fact, the deepest levels of a Master/sub relationship have nothing to do with sex at all. The elements of BDSM – trust, obedience, offering sacrifice, service, and connection – make it a practice of the soul.

In order to take you to the edge and encourage you to always expand your limits a Master must reach deep into the core of your psyche. The experience of having a woman open herself so fully, without hesitation, changes a Master's inner nature, making him strong and loving at the same time.

To find a partner able to get that intensely entrenched into your mind, body and spirit is to have a rare jewel indeed. As the Master's submissive, you have great value to him, and he is worth much to you.

In a world where so many things are destructive, disappointing, or come with hidden strings your desire to give and not take, to serve and not demand, to trust and not fear, to share and not hide places you on a pinnacle in your Master's experience. When you bow before him, wearing his collar as a signal to the entire world that you belong to this man – not because you were forced but because you found him worthy to bestow your very being to his will – you bring him great honor.

Never underestimate the power of the ability to give pleasure and to make his happiness your pleasure. There are none as dear to us as those who please us because of their will to do so.

As a joined couple, Master and sub, you create a new entity; a reality which requires both of you for it to exist. You are a highly valued woman never to be taken for granted because you give the Master the one thing no one else in the world can give. You make him complete.

Likewise, his training, his love, his security, and his strength complete you also. As such, you will learn to regard yourself as the Master's treasure and he yours. When you see each other in this way, the soul joining that occurs makes your relationship rare and beautiful.

3. Proper Names

Names not only tell people who we are, they also reveal our relationship, status and what happens to be going on at a certain time. When your mother calls you by your full name, you know you are in trouble. Someone trying to keep you at a professional distance may call you by your title (Mrs. Miss. Ms. Dr.) and your last name as way of being respectful and not too familiar.

A friend may call you by your first name or a nickname that has developed between the two of you. A parent sometimes calls you "Angel" or "Sweetie" to reveal their affection for you. Much in the same way, you will establish yourself as a slave in training by the names you are called, and the names you call others.

The first job in training is to strip away as much of your prior social conditioning as possible to give you space to create a new reality as your Master's property. As such it is highly unlikely your Master will call you by your given first name or a last name whatsoever.

Depending on the method your Master chooses to use, he may refer to you by a term that is degrading or vulgar until you are stripped of your own ego shell and molded into the form you desire.

Your Master may refer to you as "slave" or "sub" along with your name, such as "Slave kate" or "Sub mary." However, most of the time he is likely to just call you by a term more descriptive of your role than your persona. Words such as "slave", "sub", "girl", "you" will become your name for a time. He will tell you which name suits him and you will answer to it at all times until it becomes second nature.

If you are in a part of training that emphasizes the sexual nature of your service he may refer to you in sexual terms. He may call you "slut," "whore," "cunt," or "cock slave," as a way of helping you acclimate to your sexual identity.

In time, as training proceeds the names will change to names reflecting the value you hold for his heart. Then you may be known as "Master's angel," "Little one," or "Beloved."

The one name you can be called at any time through the process is the one you cannot be given. It must be earned. That name is "Good girl" and the thrill you get in your heart when he says it makes all the other names worthwhile.

You do not get to choose what you call him. He will instruct you on how you should address him at all times. In most protocol situations a sub may never use the Master's given or first name during service. You may call him "Master," "Sir," or "My Lord" but you never call him "Brian", "Honey" or by a nickname he has not chosen.

Names have the power to help us understand, honor and communicate who we are. As such, you always want to refer to your Master by the proper term and no other.

Your Master will also instruct you in the ways you should communicate to others. Since other men, even if they are Doms, are not your Master, you would not call them Master. You would call them, "Sir" or refer to them as "Master Jim" or as another's slave's master such as "Slave Kate's Master."

You would never answer another Dom without using "Sir" or another term of respect. In sub-to-sub communication first names are generally used if all subs are seen at an equal level. Your Master may also ask you to refer to all men respectfully, such as saying "Thank you, Sir," to the mailman or a store clerk.

What we call people changes how we see them and see ourselves, thus proper names are a primary part of training.

4. Proper Language

Just as the proper name helps you reframe the way you understand yourself and the world around you, using the proper form of language also plays a role in helping you enjoy and thrive in your position.

A sub should never use language that expresses personal power, equality of status, or unfairly manipulates a situation. You would never say phrases such as "I want" or "I think" or "I say it's like this." Those phrases put the emphasis back on the will of the sub and not in deference to the Master.

A sub should say "I would like" or "I ask" instead. If your Master asks for your opinion you would say "I would like to suggest we see a movie", not "I want to see a movie" or "I think we should see a movie." Remember, when your Master asks for your opinion, it is a gift to you and you should respond with gratitude.

Foul language is powerful. That's why we say those words when someone cuts us off on the freeway. They have power and they make us feel more powerful. As such, a sub should never use foul language voluntarily or in any situation. A sub's speech should be plain, demur and reflect a disciplined nature and tongue.

Your Master may wash your mouth with soap or devise another punishment for you if your language reflects poor deportment or brings more power to you than is appropriate.

There are times when a Master may ask you to use poor language during a training or sexual session. If he asks you to talk dirty to him, or repeat phrases such as "I am your slut" or "I am your fuck toy, I was made to be fucked by you," then obviously it is alright to do so. However, in everyday communication the classier a slave keeps her language, the better for her and her Master.

5. Proper Clothing

When you agreed to submit your body to your Master one of the things you gave him the right/responsibility to do is dress you. Like the rest of your life, there will be different types of acceptable attire depending on the situation and the scene your Master wants to set before you.

Clothing, or lack thereof, will differ based on the public/private aspect as well as the purpose/pleasure component. However, the one item that is the most important (even when you are not wearing it) is your collar.

The collar is an item of great value to a submissive and a pride to her Master. The collar shows your level of commitment and the power of your offering. It is a reminder to you of the strength and ownership your Master has and a reinforcement of your identity as his. It is evidence to all others who see it that you are an owned being and not your own person. It shows the power of the relationship you have, and undeniable bond between you and your Master.

Your Master will pick out your collar and you may go through several while in training. To start, many Masters choose a common dog collar. If it is possible, ask your Master if you may go with him to buy it. The trip to the pet shop to get it, and trying it on in public, is one of the most intense and sexually arousing moments a Master and slave can have early in the process.

If your Master opts to start you off with a fancier training collar, there are many leather and fetish shops online that can supply anything he needs, from simple leather to studded and styled. The moment he puts that collar around your neck and buckles it is a sacred, important initiation for you as a submissive.

Because many people cannot go to work or out in society with wearing a dog collar, your Master will also gift you with a "symbolic collar" to wear in public so the vanilla world won't be aware of your status. Some Masters wait until you've finished the training phase and gift you with the collar at a formal ceremony; others want you in your public collar as soon as possible.

Usually the public collar is a necklace (sometimes bracelet) with a lock, heart or other meaningful symbol of your submission. Wear it proudly and enjoy the connection to your Master at all times.

Apart from the collar, a submissive will generally be kept naked during training when inside the house. Nudity helps create a sense of openness to your Master as you offer all of your parts without any barrier for his visual and personal pleasure. It's also a very practical thing during training because there will be a lot of spanking, bondage, and sex during the process so this will reduce the time it takes to prepare for a few swats or instant service.

One of the great benefits of submission is the chance for you to gather body esteem often denied to women by society, as the focus on your body is present and positive. Corsets or other sexual attire may be required for play parties or socializing with other Doms/subs.

For dress in public your Master may choose your clothing each day or may give you the freedom to dress yourself as long as the clothing is approved. At any time, if a Master says he does not like what you are wearing, he has the right to tell you to change. A wise Master understands if you have to dress for work a certain way, but if he wants you in a dress to go to the grocery store, it is your job to comply.

Sometimes when you will be in public in a casual setting (a movie, etc.) he may tell you he doesn't want you to wear underwear, so that he may play with you during your time together. Underwear is almost always a "by permission only" article of clothing for a sub.

6. Proper Graces

The focus of a submissive woman's pleasure is to ensure that she is providing her Master pleasure in all ways. Everything you do is a reflection on your Master and his training. A slave who is awkward, loud, rude, or sloppy does not bring pride and pleasure to her master and may find herself on the unhappy end of the strap if her deportment doesn't improve.

A submissive woman should be a lady, in every way, and employ all the social graces to ensure her Master's dignity and comfort.

Subs should always be neat. When you come home from work or a public setting and you are taking your clothes off to be properly naked before your Master for the rest of the evening, make sure to hang or fold your clothing neatly, or deposit in the laundry basket for later washing.

If your Master removes your clothes and throws them on the floor, wait until your pleasure together is finished, but as he sleeps or when possible, pick up your clothing and put them in a proper place.

A good submissive is an orderly one. If you don't take care of your surroundings, how can you be trusted to care for your Master?

The same holds true for domestic and sexual service. If you bring your Master a drink, don't just plunk it down on the table. Kneel before him and offer it to him. If he directs you to set it on the table, do so gently so as not to disturb him.

Walk softly, don't stomp around. Most importantly, use a soft and pliant vocal tone. No one enjoys a submissive who barks statements with a rough or sarcastic flavor. When you are allowed to speak, do so slowly, lowly and gently.

7. Proper Postures

There are several different acceptable "basic postures" for a submissive/slave and your Master will train you very early which one he prefers as your default posture and in what settings other postures will be appropriately used.

The most basic posture of greeting or waiting is kneeling. A submissive should kneel with her calves flat on the ground, her bottom resting on her heels. You should have your back straight, your legs slightly apart, and your open hands on top of your thighs.

Your gaze should be at the floor in front of you, or looking straight ahead, never looking up at the Master unless he guides your eyes in that direction. The openness of the legs and hands shows your Master you are open and ready for service of any kind.

The other posture thought of as the default submissive posture, particularly if you are offering sexual service at that time, is "face down, ass up." A static genuflecting posture, this shows your sexual submission by exposing your genitals in a direct way. It also has the benefit of showing your identity (your face) is in the lower position while your Master's pleasure is in the upper position.

The best way to gracefully assume this posture is to get on your hands and knees, then quickly bend your arms to lower your face to the carpet while sticking your bottom up in the air, legs parted as much as possible.

If you have strong core muscles and a good back, you can extend your arms out in front of your head as a supplicating gesture. On the other hand, if you don't have a good back, your Master may allow you to rest on your elbows and knees, giving your spine more support. Like all positions, the longer you stay in this position, the more natural and comfortable it will begin to feel.

For serving a dinner, the Master may ask you to take a servant's stance beside the table as he and his guests eat. This would involve you standing straight, legs comfortably apart, hands at your side or behind your back, face forward (so you can watch your guests to see if there is anything needed).

For a causal day at home, your Master may want you lying flat on the floor under his feet, kneeling beside him, or laying on the couch with your face in his lap providing some pleasure while he enjoys the game. Men are visual creatures so he will almost always want you on display in the room with him so he can look at your body and enjoy you.

There are a lot of postures you will be asked to assume, and there are also postures that a sub without permission must NEVER do. A submissive woman should never place her arms or hands in any way that blocks off a part of her body. Do not put your hands in front of your genitals or cross your arms over your chest (a communication and body blocking stance).

A sub should never sit with her legs closed or crossed unless you are in public and have permission. A sub should never look directly at her Master without his permission. You will spend a lot of time in silence, so your body is the best way you have to communicate your love and devotion to his pleasure.

8. The Value of Silence

One of the major differences between online submission and real-time experiences is the amount of downtime and silence involved. In online submission you are plugged in and active via email or chat during your time with your Master. You don't sit naked in front of a computer staring at a blank screen while he watches a baseball game or reads a book.

On the other hand, real life experiences often come with a lot of waiting, introspection and silence. It is actually a wonderful chance for you to slow down, think and process your life as a submissive. With time and practice you will learn to value it. You will also learn the many ways you can communicate without speaking.

If your Master asks you to wait by the door to greet him when he comes home, don't play on the computer or do chores until the second he pulls into the driveway, then run to the door and kneel. There is nothing appealing about a sweating, panting slave who smells like Pine Sol.

Make sure to get in your position at least fifteen minutes prior to his expected arrival. What are you going to do with all that time? Think. Pray. Enjoy. Rest. Imagine the rest of your night. Most importantly, let yourself build up anticipation for when you see him. In a world full of constant access, cell phones and noise the quiet time you have before your Master arrives is a real gift.

A submissive should never speak until they are spoken to or have asked permission to speak. Your voice is part of what you have given to your Master. He may want to engage in a conversation with you about your day, in which case you will talk plenty, or he may want to just enjoy the quiet with you by his side.

If there is something you need to say or ask, then softly ask for permission to speak. If he grants it, then you may ask your question or make your comment. If he does not, then return to silence.

During the training period the silence will seem prolonged, painful and, well…boring. We live in a run around world where silence, patience and peace are hard to find. Some Masters only allow their submissive to use three phrases during training: "Yes Sir," "Please Sir," and "Thank you, Sir."

In training the idea of saying "No Sir" is never going to happen. Subs do not say "no." However, as your training evolves you will find you Master lets you be more participative in the process and you enjoy the sanity and tranquility of service.

9. Asking Permission

The Master in the relationship has the responsibility of making the decisions. His dominance frees you from those concerns. However, when you have a partner who has gifted you by making your decisions, you have the obligation to respect and allow him to do that. Permission plays a very important role in everything you will do, say, eat, wear, and plan.

The primary rule for submissive women in a BDSM relationship is this: Never tell, always ask. A sub should never put herself in any kind of power position over the Master where she "tells" him something. She is the receiver. He is the giver.

If there is something you want to do or say, you must ask your Master politely for permission. Hence, you would never say to your Master, "I am going to the store" or "I need to go to the store." You would ask, "May I go to the store, Sir?"

During training, which is generally stricter than daily life, permission isn't just about what you want to say or what you can wear. Permission is about everything. You will need to ask your Master for permission to leave the room, enter the room, and to go to the bathroom.

Even if you ask permission to leave the room, if you are going to the bathroom make sure to ask specific permission to do that. If the answer is no, then you will have to wait. During training, Masters are trying to teach you the understanding that they are in charge of all your bodily functions, and as a result will be the deciding factor in your bathroom habits.

Sexuality is another area permission will become an important concept. Never touch your Master or take him into your mouth without his expressed permission. If he teaches you there is a signal (a snap of the finger or pat on the head) that tells you it's okay to take him in your mouth, follow that. However, even if he is standing with his cock in front of your mouth, look up or ask for permission, don't just assume you have the right to touch him. That also goes for your own body.

Never masturbate or touch yourself in a sexual way without his consent or presence. Your pleasure is not supposed to be separate from his pleasure. He may ask you to masturbate while he watches you for his pleasure or he may reward you with allowing you a private orgasm of your own. However, those are his choices, not yours.

One of the very first lessons you will learn during the sexual portion of your training is that you do not have the right to orgasm without his permission. When you feel yourself nearing the inevitable release, you must ask him for permission to experience orgasm.

If you are in a gag or not allowed to speak you can use your body, hands or eye movement to ask. However, never climax without his permission or you will find yourself in a chastity belt or experiencing celibacy and frustration as a punishment for a long time.

10. Attentiveness

One of the reasons a Master/submissive relationship has such great depth and intensity is because you are focused on each other and not your own issues, stuff or distractions. Instead of sitting down at night and pouring yourself into a book, website, or TV show, you are thinking about pleasing and being present with one another. Attentiveness is one of the most attractive things in the day-to-day life of a submissive and her Master.

You must ensure your Master never has a need that goes unmet as long as it is something you can fulfill. Never let your Master be hungry, thirsty or want for something. Keep an eye on his glass and when he is nearly finished ask him if he would like some more.

When he is finished eating ask for permission to take his plate or clear the table. Make sure the space in front of him is clean. If you know he is going to watch TV, find the remote and kneel before him, handing it to him or leave it by his chair so it is available.

The less effort he has to put into the small things of life, the more energy he will have to pay attention to you and be present with you.

Once you know your Master's preferences for food, drink, habits or hobbies make sure he doesn't have to ask you for things. If you help him in the garage, learn the names of the tools (or what he calls them) so you can hand him the right thing when he asks for it.

If he is going to work set up his lunch or briefcase and have everything ready for him to walk out the door. If you are busy getting ready for work as well, set everything up the night before.

Your Master may grant you permission to play on the Internet, do some work at home (for example – if you are a teacher and need to grade papers), or watch a show. When those times occur make sure you are still attentive to your Master in case a need arises. If you're playing a game online, make sure it's one you can stop or pause so that you can get him something to drink or meet his need.

Under no circumstances should you expect your Master to wait on you to finish a level, come to the end of a page, or get to a commercial. That defeats the whole purpose of a couple enjoying the BDSM life.

As you focus on him, you will also learn his moods and desires. If you notice he is edgy and may like something to help him relax, make sure he knows you are wanting and available for that. If you have displeased him and were punished but he still seems out of sorts, ask for permission to do something to help make things better. As your Master, he will do the same for you.

Being entwined in each other's moods and needs is very much at the heart of a couple where submission is a component. Your Master should never have to "get your attention." It should always be his.

11. Gratitude

Submission is a life change that doesn't just alter the way you dress, act and relate to one another. In the long term, it actually changes your perspective on life. One of the greatest gifts training as a submissive/slave will teach you is the gift of gratitude.

You will become thankful for the smallest things and the largest surprises. You won't be taking things for granted anymore and you won't have a list of expectations, but a list of joys you are thankful to receive. In many ways submission is the perfect antidote to our selfish, greedy social culture.

Be thankful for everything your submission brings to you through the day. If the Master gives you chores to do, thank him for the privilege of serving him that way. There is a lot of down time in submission. Activity gives you a chance to add variety to your moment. Once you've been sitting at his feet staring off into the distance for most of the afternoon, a chance to get up, get him some tea or do the dishes will seem like a vacation. More than that, being thankful for the tasks he assigns you is a way of acknowledging to him that his pleasure is your pleasure and you love to meet his needs.

If the Master grants anything you ask – permission to leave the room, a chance to eat some lunch, the ability to climax – make sure to always respond with, "Thank you, Master."

It is also important that you not thank your Master only for the good things, but for the harsh things as well. Training involves a lot of punishment and correction. The Master punishes you in order to teach you the best way to do things, and help you feel the accomplishment of learning and growing. The Master takes time away from his pleasure to correct you and uses his energy to teach you.

Submissive partners tend to see training as a time when they can't do anything right and they have to endure it. However, the reality is also that training is a time when the Master has to be hyper-vigilant, responsive and corrective. Training can be hard on a sub (particularly her behind) but it is equally exhausting and challenging for her Master. Thank him for his spankings, his corrections, his lectures and for giving you another chance to learn.

The more you thank your Master for the punishments and guidance he gives you, the more firmly entrenched in his love and power you will become. You will begin to see his punishments as a gift to you and a way of making you a stronger couple. In all the ways you will grow in grace through your training, developing a heart full of gratitude is one of the best.

12. Submitting Your Body for Inspection

You are his. Your mind is his. Your time is his. Your talents are his. Your body is his. As such, your body is the object of submission to which he will pay the most attention. You must always keep your body clean, nude, presentable and open for his inspection in any way.

When your Master looks at you, he smiles with the knowledge that he owns everything he sees, and he will want to see it all. Every day in every way, your body will be open for inspection.

Almost all Masters require their submissive partners to be fully shaved in the pubic area. Genital hair is considered an offensive covering of the Master's property and he will not want to see it.

In training he may want to shave you himself for the first time as a sign of him taking possession of his property. After that time, you will be responsible to keep yourself shaved and smooth for the Master. That means no stubble.

If you do not wax or use laser removal, it is best to shave every day or every other day. For one thing, it keeps the itch of re-growing hair from happening. The other benefit is there is not stubble or stray hair to cause the Master displeasure and discomfort.

You should not expect privacy of any kind for any action during your training. You will likely be told to use the bathroom with the door open, as well as shower or bathe that way. You will sleep naked, either on the floor beside the Master's bed or, if you are a lucky sub, in bed with your Master. Your legs should always be slightly open and in the house you will wear nothing but your collar.

If your Master takes you to a munch, play party or BDSM conference you may be required to stand with your legs open, arms out and allow other Masters to touch your body, including inserting his fingers into your vaginal lips.

When your Master puts you on display for another's inspection, he is presenting you as a matter of pride and ownership. You should feel honored that he lets another Dom touch you and inspect the quality of his submissive.

Always make sure you are prepared for that eventuality and be clean and ready. If it is your monthly cycle, make sure your Master understands that ahead of time so there are no awkward moments.

In public or in private, your body must not only be available for your Master's eyes, touch and tongue, but it must be pleasing as well. Take care of fingernails, toenails, body hair, ear wax or any other issue that may prove less than desirable for your Master. You always want to be allowed to look into his eyes and see the glow of pride that says, "This woman is mine."

13. Submitting Your Body for Correction.

Punishment and correction are primary tools that will be used throughout training and your relationship. Not every spanking, bondage event or pain you experience will be because of punishment. Many times your Master may spank you for pleasure or to enjoy a light red hue on your naked cheeks as a visual reminder of your submission to him. However, when you step out of your defined place as a submissive woman, you will be corrected, quickly and painfully.

The type of correction your Master might choose differs depending on the offense and the level of correction required. It will likely be a combination of a lecture or lesson, a physical punishment, a consequence and a chance for an apology.

The physical punishment may be as small as an Over-the-Knee (OTK) spanking, or a lashing with a single tail whip. It can be as quick as a slap in the face, or you may endure hours of being bound in an uncomfortable position with a plug in your ass and binder clips on your nipples.

It all depends on what your Master thinks is required for you to learn. However, you will learn to submit your body for correction no matter what that entails.

Depending on your experience with physical punishment prior to training, your Master will probably start you out with hand spankings, adding a hairbrush, paddle or belt into the mix as time goes by. The important thing is to bend over for your spanking without hesitation.

If he sits down and pats his lap for you to go OTK, lean over quickly, placing your hands on the floor or bed in front of you. It is very important that once you are in position you voluntarily raise your rear for his first hit. Don't make him shift his legs around or pull you upward. Raise your hips to show him you are willing to submit to his correction and you do so with a full heart.

If his punishment involves tying or bondage, keep your arms/hands/legs in the position he requires for as long as it takes him to tie you. Some bondage positions and knots can take anywhere from 5 to 25 minutes to secure. If he intends to punish your breasts by either slapping or clamping, hold them up for him or stick them out to show your desire for his lessons.

Inevitably, the pain is going to take over and you will lose control of your body parts. Your legs are going to start swinging or you may flinch or move back from a painful moment. However, the more you recover from those times and show him you are willing and desiring for him to correct you, the more you will please him.

Submissives are forbidden at all times to cover or shield their body from their Master's correction. If you are enduring a spanking and reach back to cover your cheeks with your hands to stop the blows, you have committed an offense possibly worse than whatever you did to earn the spanking. Grip the bedspread, carpet or chair legs if you have to, but never put your hands back to attempt to stop the spanking.

In the same way, you must not stop the punishment on your own accord. Early in training the Master will likely give you a safe word so he can get to know you and your pain limits. However, rarely will that word be used in punishment situations (they are supposed to hurt).

If there is something unbearable happening, attempt to communicate that to your Master respectfully. Never reach up and pull the clamps off or just stand up and get off his lap without permission. It shows a terrible lack of respect for your Master.

No one likes being punished for doing something wrong. That's what motivates us to do things right. Your Master, also, gets less pleasure from having to correct you. If he just wanted to spank you for fun, he could do that. Having to correct your behavior is a chore to him and a responsibility he has undertaken. He would much rather be thinking up kinky fun for you both to share than punishing you.

Submitting your body, without bargaining, arguing, or hesitation is the best way to show him that you are both on the same page.

14. Submitting Your Body for Ownership

Your collar is the ultimate symbol of your submission, but there are other ways your Master will choose to reinforce his ownership of your body. The most likely will be maintenance spankings.

A maintenance spanking is a spanking your Master administers to you not because you have done something wrong, but just as a reminder that you are his. They are usually hand or paddle spankings administered on the bare behind so that some pinkness lasts about an hour or two.

In training that can become a ritual and you may receive several spankings a day in order to keep your bottom in a constant state of redness. For submissive women who work outside the home, Masters will often administer a harder maintenance spanking before you leave for work, or give you one when you come home to get you back into the swing of things.

Your Master may give you a collar, ring or bracelet for you to wear in public as a sign of his ownership. In a casual public setting, such as out to dinner, a movie, etc., he may tell you to wear a butt plug anally or a remote egg vibrator inside your vagina to ensure his presence in your thoughts and body during your time out around town. He will tell you how to cut your hair, polish your nails, dress and eat. All of these are ways you submit to the reality of his ownership of your body.

Sexually he may reinforce ownership by using lipstick or marker to write on your body. If you are going through humiliation training, he may choose to write words like "slut," "Daddy's whore," or "fucktoy" on you and take you to a play party or take pictures of you in that state to put on a fetish website.

Submitting yourself to such treatment can be hard at first. However, the pleasure he gets from owning you and your commitment to his ownership will soon replace any sense of dread with joy and fulfillment.

15. Submitting Your Body for Sexual Service

When couples in vanilla relationships hear about a couple practicing BDSM or in a Master/submissive relationship they tend to think it is all about sex. They couldn't be more wrong.

The core of the relationship is about trust, sacrifice, depth of commitment and journeying together. Sex isn't what defines the relationship. However, sex is a big part of it. If you are giving yourself to someone intimately, then sex is the way to best experience that intimate reality.

As a submissive you will give your body to your Master for sexual service. There is so much to learn (and unlearn from cultural myths and social roles) that you will go through specific sexual training as well as your general training as a submissive.

You will spend a large amount of time learning how to use your body to please your Master, and how to let go of your resistance to allow your body to be used by your Master. Your Master will listen to your sexual history then create a series of goals for you to expand your limits and grow together as a couple.

The reason you can't "just do what you've always done" is to provide you with experiences you can have together so you share more than sex acts – you share a sexual journey. All of your body belongs to your Master for training and use, but the focus will largely fall into three general categories.

16. Submitting Your Mouth for Your Master's Use

Oral dominance is one of the first ways your Master will establish rule over your body. You will be expected to provide oral sex at any time, under any amount of scrutiny at a moment's notice.

At first your Master will work with you on giving a basic blow job, working toward the goal of being able to take the full length of his penis into your mouth and throat. He will also instruct you to gently suck and lick his testicles.

Although he may choose, on occasion, to withdraw his penis and ejaculate on your face or breasts as a sign of ownership, most of the time he will expect you to swallow his ejaculate, preferably not spilling any out of your mouth.

If you have trouble swallowing, your Master will use training techniques to get you more used to the taste of him, including ejaculating onto a plate or bowl and having you eat it, or ejaculating in the front of your mouth and making you hold it there while the taste permeates your consciousness.

Eventually, use of your mouth will broaden to include training you to simply hold his cock in your mouth for long periods of time, gently kissing or licking it. This will most often be the case when he is focused on something else (work, watching TV) and he just wants you to provide comfort or attention to his cock.

You will also be trained to provide anilingus – the practice of licking or rimming his anus with your tongue. Any part of his body will likely end up in your mouth. You will lick his feet, suck his fingers and give him a myriad of pleasurable feelings through your oral submission.

17. Submitting Your Vagina for Your Master's Use

That's the least shocking concept, but also the most profound. When you open yourself up to your Master, you are taking him inside your body. That intimacy should always be understood and available to your Master.

In the earliest stages of training your Master will frequently check you for wetness and arousal. You want to be internally lubricated and show yourself to be excited for him to take you.

Normally, between the nudity of submission and the overwhelming power of newness in training, it won't be very hard for him to find you wet. If you do find yourself struggling to show arousal, create a series of fantasies, memories or sexy thoughts you run through your mind that will help begin the self-lubricating process.

Your master will also use dildos and vibrators as part of your sexual submission. He may want you to carry the sensation of being "filled" while you do something in the house, or keep your sexual submission readily in your mind.

As your journey progresses he may use things like ginger jelly to provide stinging sensations, or spank or whip your labia with a riding crop as a form of both sex and/or discipline.

The other way you will encounter vaginal submission isn't when he uses you, but when he chooses not to use you. As a form of discipline or control training, it is not uncommon for a Master to put his submissive through a period of chastity.

There are many online retailers that sell actual chastity belts that can be worn under clothing. Locking your vagina behind a metal plate and literally handing your Master the key to your sex is a powerfully advanced form of submission. Others may use restrictions on sexuality without the formal chastity device, as a part of training.

18. Submitting Your Ass for Sexual Service

This area tends to require more training than the other two because many people come into a relationship with little or no anal sex experience. That makes the anus one of the prime targets for your Master early in training.

When you submit to your Master no place is private and no hole is barred. If you are completely new to anal submission, your Master may start you off with a series of butt plugs as a training tool. These plugs come in a set, increasing in size and shape. He will start you off by inserting the smallest one and have you wear that for a certain amount of time each day until you are used to the feeling. Over time, he will use larger plugs until you are ready for his penis.

After training you can still expect to wear an anal plug some of the time. If you have a job that affords accommodating attire, he may require you to insert it or wear it for some time during work to remind you of his ownership when you are not at home.

If you attend a dinner or movie, your Master may put a remote egg vibrator inside a plug and activate it from time to time during the event just to send you a little thrill that your Master is thinking about you.

Sometimes a plug with prongs or with a bulb in the base area (where the sphincters are) will be used during a spanking as a form of punishment.

The goal of all this training is that you will, without hesitance, argument, fear or question, provide your Master any kind of sexual service he desires to share with you. This submission will provide you tremendous pleasure as well. Your body will be luxuriated in attention, appreciated and satisfied along with your relationship.

Section II: How You Will Learn It

Now that you've seen all the things you will learn, it's time to look at how you will learn them.

19. Through Obedience

Modern wedding ceremonies may have taken the word "obey" out of their liturgy, but it is front and center in understanding a Master/submissive relationship. As a woman offering the gift of submission to your Master you accept the prime responsibility to obey him in all things. That sounds really pretty until you realize how little we obey anyone or anything in our vanilla lives. We have trouble obeying the speed limit, which is a law enforced by authority. How much harder is it to obey every command from your lover clearly and correctly?

For obedience training, your Master will establish a set of rules and goals you will be expected to live by and accomplish. Some will be common sense and some will stretch your limits. Any deviation from the rules or the standard of excellence he sets for you will be met with swift punishment and correction.

For example, if your car is prone to get a little messy due to eating on the way to work or leaving papers in the back seat, your Master may tell you that you are to keep your car perfectly clean. A few weeks later he may inspect it in the morning and find an empty soda can or piece of junk mail you forgot to throw away. He will call you out to look at what he found and have you clean up the mess immediately. He will then talk to you about why it is important to keep your car clean and remind you it is his expectation.

Then he will give you a hard spanking with a belt that is a discipline (pain based) spanking, not an erotic (pleasure based) spanking. After that, he may assign a consequence such as making you walk to the post office, or ride with a co-worker for a week to impress upon you the privilege of having a car. Finally, he will allow you to thank him for his correction and apologize for the offense to be forgiven.

What does the state of your car have to do with your relationship? Everything. Because the issue is obedience. Throughout training your Master will set up tests, rules, and expectations for you. He will want to see you follow his directions. If he snaps his fingers for you to provide him oral pleasure he will want to see you drop to your knees immediately and embrace him. Over time, the tests will fade away and the rules and ideas that frame your normal everyday life will take hold.

20. Through Objectification

Not all Masters use this tool as part of a training regimen however, many find it to be helpful for women who have power positions at work or have never been in a power exchange relationship before. Objectification involves spending time treating the submissive partner as if she were an object or servant without feelings or recourse. It is never done as the only part of training and your Master will explain the benefits of objectification to you as well as the parameters of the exercise.

Sometimes objectification is done by placing the submissive in the room as an object – bent over to be a table upon which the Master sets his drink or lined up against the wall holding a tray with some flowers as an ornamental decoration while the Master goes about his business. If you are in a polyamorous relationship where the Master has more than one submissive, he may use you to hold drinks and watch as he sexually enjoys another submissive.

Objectification is also used at play parties where submissive partners are dressed as serving girls with trays or other devices strapped onto their bodies and used to provide refreshments for the guests. Guests have the right to touch or tease the servant as they desire. At play parties of a more sexual nature a submissive may be put into a pleasure swing to be used by anyone at the party as a sort of "party favor."

For periods where objectification is the method of training, the Master will refer to you as "it" and regard you casually, as if you were a piece of the surrounding environment.

The purpose of objectification is to strip away the ego and the self-obsession that often attaches to us in the larger culture. For a submissive woman who is used to the world being "all about her," the practice of objectifying her frees her from the need to be the center of attention so the focus can return to the couple at large.

Women who have powerful jobs where they carry a large amount of responsibility often find freedom and release in objectification. They can retreat into the background and not be the focus of anything. A little time as an anonymous being is like taking a vacation from the weight of the world.

21. Through Humiliation

While not all Masters employ specific objectification in training, all Masters will use some form of humiliation as part of the learning process. Your gut reaction to the word "humiliation" may be very negative. Remember, the word is connected to the same root as the word "humility" and that is the ultimate goal of humiliating experiences.

When you think about it, almost everything that attracts you to BDSM has a humiliating or humbling component to it. A grown woman taking off her underpants and bending over a man's lap for a bare bottom spanking isn't just a fetish. It is rooted in the shame of the stripping down and the embarrassment that you are receiving the type of punishment a child gets.

This humiliation is often further exaggerated by the practice of "corner time" where the submissive woman is sent to stand with her nose in the corner and her bare red bottom on display so she can think about and reflect on the humbling situation.

If you travel out of town or with another Master/submissive couple, your Master may spank you until you are very red, put you in a corner with your panties down and call for room service to bring a tray into the room, or invite the other couple to dine while you are on display. Experiences like that have a sexual component that builds excitement and obedience at the same time.

Sometimes humiliation may be a part of the consequences of your correction. For example, let's say you checked out a library book and kept it far past the deadline. Your Master corrects you for the procrastination and gives you a good, hard spanking. He then takes you to the library and instructs you to pay the fine and apologize to the librarian for keeping the book out so long.

If he wants to make the lesson even more memorable, he may instruct you to tell the librarian that you were spanked for keeping the book out. That kind of awkward moment will certainly correct the behavior in the future.

Wise Masters know where the boundaries of that kind of training exist and would not put an unsuspecting person in too much of an awkward situation. However, humiliation training will almost always find its way into the corrective and instructive moments of your relationship.

If you should insult or resist another Master, it is highly likely your Master will allow him to spank you or correct you in front of the group.

As training progresses and your natural submissive nature takes over, you will find purposeful humiliation to play less of a role in your relationship because your Master will not need to use it as much. At that point it becomes something you have as a tool for sexual pleasure and fun.

22. By Repetition And Ritual

If practice makes perfect, then by the time your Master is ready to transition you from training to daily service you will be as close to perfect as a human can get. Repetition is a mainstay of your training time. You will do specific things a certain way over and over again. This both ensures you will learn to do things the way that pleases your Master best, and your submission makes its way into your subconscious thought.

Rituals play a very important role in helping you reach into that inner clay of who you are and mold it into a happy, satisfying submissive life. You will be instructed to bow, kneel or respond in unique ways every time your Master enters the room so the environment is set for your submission.

You may be asked to repeat phrases over and over again. It is common for a Master to lay his submissive on the bed naked and touch each of her body parts, having her repeat things like , "That is your mouth, Master. " "Those are your breasts, Master." "That is your ass, Master." This repetition reinforces the idea that you are his for both of you to understand.

If your Master tells you to set the table a certain way, or lick the back of his shaft before mouthing the tip of his penis, you will do it that way every time until the practice becomes second nature. If you make a mistake or require correction you can be sure the Master will have you repeat the task over and over.

Many rituals you undergo during your training as a submissive are beautiful and will hold a very special place in your memory. The first time he collars you or the ceremony where he removes your training collar and gives you a permanent one are joys most of the world will never understand. When you please him and he looks at you and says, "Good girl" the feeling of those words will swell your heart with joy.

23. By Affection

Not everything in training is harsh, objectifying or painful. A lot of the time your training and challenges will be interspersed with moments of sincere affection and absolute love. Your Master will run his hands through your hair and across your body. He will tell you how beautiful you are in his eyes. He will be thankful and nurturing as you serve him.

After the punishment he will engage in aftercare, holding you and applying lotion to your behind. He will encourage you to keep trying, and keep learning. Many submissive women comfort themselves through the pain of punishment with thoughts of the love and affirmation that will come afterward.

A wise Master never withdraws affection as a form of punishment or correction. He will, instead, punish with a stern hand and then shower you with praise for your endurance and desire to do better. Many nights will be made of long, touching loving sessions where you are connected – Master and sub – physically while you watch a show or play a game.

His pride in you will be apparent for all to see. His care for you will uplift your spirit and esteem. Your joining, where you are focused on each other and not the distractions and pressures of society, will be deep, sustaining and beautiful.

Conclusion

A healthy BDSM relationship is not something that just pops out of the box (or your computer) readymade. It takes time, trust, trial and error, failure and victory, love, laughter, and joy.

As you go through these things on the journey to become the woman you were made to be, you will be tested but you will also be proud, joyful and, perhaps for the first time in your life, you will be at peace.

Other books by Elizabeth Cramer:

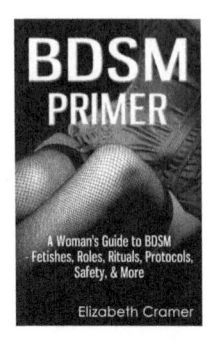

BDSM Primer - A Woman's Guide to BDSM - Fetishes, Roles, Rituals, Protocols, Safety, & More

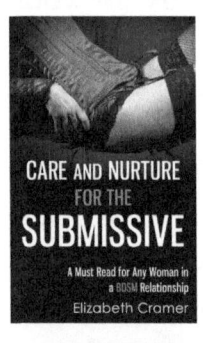

Care and Nurture for the Submissive - A Must Read for Any Woman in a BDSM Relationship

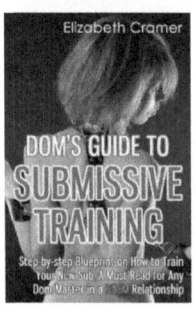

Dom's Guide To Submissive Training: Step-by-step Blueprint On How To Train Your New Sub. A Must Read For Any Dom/Master In A BDSM Relationship

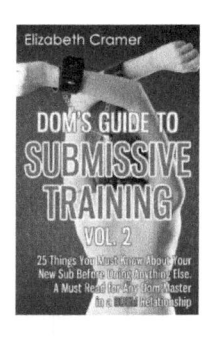

Dom's Guide To Submissive Training Vol. 2: 25 Things You Must Know About Your New Sub Before Doing Anything Else. A Must Read For Any Dom/Master In A BDSM Relationship

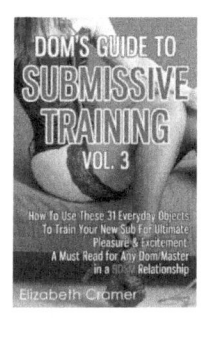

Dom's Guide To Submissive Training Vol. 3: How To Use These 31 Everyday Objects To Train Your New Sub For Ultimate Pleasure & Excitement. A Must Read For Any Dom/Master In A BDSM Relationship

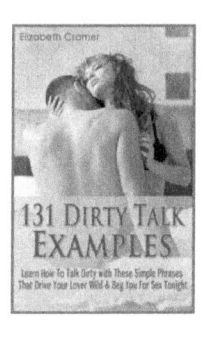

131 Dirty Talk Examples: Learn How To Talk Dirty with These Simple Phrases That Drive Your Lover Wild & Beg You For Sex Tonight

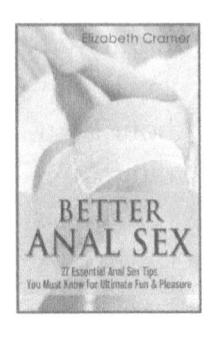

Better Anal Sex - 27 Essential Anal Sex Tips You Must Know for Ultimate Fun & Pleasure

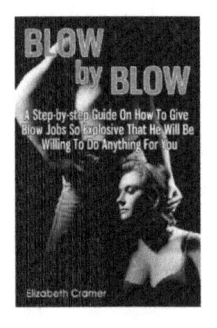

Blow By Blow - A Step-by-step Guide On How To Give Blow Jobs So Explosive That He Will Be Willing To Do Anything For You

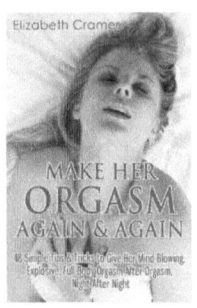

Make Her Orgasm Again and Again: 48 Simple Tips & Tricks to Give Her Mind-Blowing, Explosive, Full-Body Orgasm After Orgasm, Night After Night